Methylene Blue

The Chromatic Cure

Methylene Blue

The Chromatic Cure

A Multi-Dimensional Approach to Wellness, Methemoglobinemia, Brain Boost, Alzheimer, Mitochondria, Cancer, COVID-19 and Neurological Challenges

by Chappell Hoffmann

Copyright

Publisher's Note

Care has been taken to confirm the accuracy of the information presented and to describe generally accepted practices. However, the author, editors, and publisher are not responsible for errors or omissions or for any consequences from application of the information in this book and make no warranty, express or implied, with respect to the contents of the publication.

TABLE OF CONTENTS

PUBLISHER'S NOTE 3

INTRODUCTION 6

THE BLUEPRINT OF HEALTH 12

    THE CHROMATIC CONNECTION TO WELLNESS................................12

CONQUERING CELLULAR DISTRESS 17

    COMBATING DISEASES AND BATTLES AGAINST COVID-19 AND ALZHEIMER'S .17
    ALZHEIMER'S DISEASE SOLUTION 21

THE ANTI-AGING POTENTIALS OF METHYLENE BLUE AND SKIN
LONGEVITY...26

    HOW METHYLENE BLUE PENETRATES THE MITOCHONDRIA AND MODULATE ROS
    IN THE ELECTRON TRANSPORT CHAIN 31

METHYLENE BLUE'S POTENTIAL IN CANCER THERAPY......................34

    THE ROLE OF METHYLENE BLUE AS AN ELECTRON CARRIER AND POTENTIAL
    IMPACT ON CANCER CELLS 34
    ENHANCED PHOTODYNAMIC THERAPY EFFICACY OF METHYLENE BLUE 38

COMBATING DEPRESSION WITH METHYLENE BLUE 45

    ASSESSING THE EFFECTIVENESS OF METHYLENE BLUE IN DEPRESSION TREATMENT
   45

HEART DISEASE AND METHYLENE BLUE..52

    METHYLENE BLUE POSITIVE IMPACT ON CARDIOVASCULAR HEALTH AND
    POTENTIAL BENEFITS 52

THE CARDIOVASCULAR EPICENTER 58

PRACTICAL APPLICATIONS AND ADMINISTRATION OF METHYLENE
BLUE IN HEALTHCARE 61

METHYLENE BLUE'S POTENTIAL FOR PAIN RELIEF UNVEILED 63
METHYLENE BLUE'S CARTILAGE SAVER AND GUT GUARDIAN 67
FORMS AND DOSAGES 69
ADMINISTRATION PROTOCOLS AND CONSIDERATIONS 71

SIDE EFFECTS OF METHYLENE BLUE 75

INTRAVENOUS ROUTE (SOLUTION) 75

Introduction

Over the years, scientists have been working hard to understand and redefine what Methylene Blue is because of its incredible ability to fight various illnesses. There's one thing we all agree on, but before we delve into that, let's explore some definitions from different professionals!

Methylene Blue is a type of organic chloride salt with 3,7-bis (dimethylamino) phenothiazin-5-ium as the counterion. It's commonly used as a dye but also possesses antioxidant, antimalarial, antidepressant, and cardioprotective properties.

It acts as an inhibitor for processes like monoamine oxidase and cholinesterase, functions as an acid-base indicator, a fluorochrome, and plays roles in histology, guanylate cyclase inhibition, and more. Simply put, it contains a compound called 3,7-bis (dimethylamino) phenothiazin-5-ium.

Methylene Blue acts as an oxidation-reduction agent. The FDA has approved its intravenous form for treating acquired methemoglobinemia in both pediatric and adult patients. Historically, it was widely used in Africa to treat malaria, but its popularity waned with the introduction of drugs like chloroquine. Researchers are also exploring its potential as a urinary tract antiseptic, inclusively it's being studied as an inhibitor of Tau protein aggregation, showing promise for Alzheimer's disease treatment.

This synthetic basic dye stains negatively charged cell components like nucleic acids. During cancer surgery, when administered in the lymphatic bed of a tumor, it helps stain lymph nodes draining from the tumor, aiding in visualizing sentinel lymph nodes. In low doses intravenously, it can convert methemoglobin to hemoglobin.

Methylene Blue appears as dark green crystals or crystalline powder with a bronze-like luster. Its solutions in water or alcohol have a deep blue color. Beyond its staining properties, it's used as a bacteriological stain and an indicator. Notably, it inhibits guanylate cyclase and has been employed in treating cyanide poisoning and reducing levels of methemoglobin.

The significance of Methylene Blue spans various medical applications and continues to be an area of active research.

The first-time we used methylene blue as a treatment was to fight against malaria. Later on, other man-made versions like chloroquine became more popular, and methylene blue took a bit of a back seat. However, there's been recent interest in bringing it back as an antimalarial treatment.

Malaria-causing parasites, especially Plasmodium falciparum, are becoming resistant to the usual drugs used against them. That's why science is taking another look at methylene blue. In tests done with cells, methylene blue has shown to be super effective against malaria (with an IC50 of only 4 nM). Plus, when tested on animals, it seems like these parasites don't easily develop resistance to methylene blue.

This makes it a pretty promising option for fighting malaria in a world where the usual drugs might not be as effective. It looks like methylene blue could be a good solution for a problem that affects poorer areas of the world. Making 1 gram of methylene blue might cost as little as 5 US cents or even less. But before we can be sure it's a safe solution, we need to look into some reports of people having bad reactions after getting treated with methylene blue. These reactions seem to be connected to a condition called G6PD deficiency, an important enzyme in red blood cells. Screening data from Nigeria suggests that about 10% of people there have this deficiency.

Besides fighting the parasites that cause malaria, there's a thought that methylene blue could also help prevent a common problem linked to malaria called methemoglobinemia. This happens when the iron in hemoglobin changes, making it harder for the blood to carry oxygen and carbon dioxide. This can lead to a type of anemia that could be deadly. Methylene blue seems like it can help prevent this by working against the process that leads to methemoglobin production.

New studies suggest that methylene blue might also protect the brain from diseases that cause damage, like stroke and Parkinson's disease. It's really helpful in situations where cells in the brain are in danger, as it promotes the use of oxygen by the cells and reduces a process called anaerobic glycolysis. So, besides its potential in treating malaria, methylene blue could have other health benefits, especially for the brain

Methylene blue has the power to reduce the production of harmful reactive oxygen species (ROS), shielding cells from glutamate blockage, lessening the drop in mitochondrial membrane potential, and providing protection against IAA neurotoxicity, among other positive effects.

These advantages are particularly important in conditions like Alzheimer's disease, Parkinson's disease, and stroke. When compared to antipsychotic drugs like phenothiazine, methylene blue shows similar protective effects for the brain but through a different mechanism.

5

Currently, methylene blue works as a specific antioxidant for mitochondria, unlike drugs such as phenothiazine that act as free radical scavengers independently of the mitochondria.

Beyond the mentioned diseases, methylene blue can also play a role in preventing and managing brain damage related to tumors. Some treatments for solid tumors involve alkylating agents like ifosfamide, which can lead to brain damage. Methylene blue seems to help mitigate this damage, although the exact way it works isn't entirely clear. It's believed to be connected to its ability to oxidize NADH and restore mitochondrial enzymes. Since Methylene blue is a neuroprotective agent, you might wonder how it tackles the harmful effects of MS, where the protective covering of nerve fibers (myelin) in the spinal cord and/or nerves is attacked and damaged by white blood cells.

Well, in MS, the immune system makes a mistake and attacks the myelin covering nerve fibers in the central nervous system. This causes communication problems between the brain and the rest of the body, leading to various symptoms and potential damage to the nerves.

Neuroprotective agents like Methylene blue aim to shield nerve cells from harm and help them survive. Methylene blue has been looked into for its antioxidant properties and its ability to counteract oxidative stress, which is linked to various neurodegenerative conditions. While these properties may have potential benefits in protecting nerve cells, it's important to note that the specific ways in which methylene blue may work with the intricate processes involved in MS are still not completely understood.

The Blueprint of Health

The Chromatic Connection to Wellness

At its core, Methylene Blue is an organic chloride salt. The primary chemical structure consists of a phenothiazine nucleus with two dimethylamino groups (3,7-bis(dimethylamino) phenothiazin-5-ium) as the counterion. This unique arrangement is crucial to its diverse functionalities. Originally recognized as a dye, Methylene Blue has evolved beyond its coloring applications.

It exhibits antioxidant, antimalarial, and cardioprotective properties. The molecule is recognized as an inhibitor of monoamine oxidase (EC 1.4.3.4), cholinesterase (EC 3.1.1.8), and guanylate cyclase (EC 4.6.1.2). Its role as an acid-base indicator, fluorochrome, and antimicrobial agent further underscores its versatility.

The fascinating relationship between color and well-being, particularly in the context of Methylene Blue have a profound impact on our emotions, perceptions, and even our physical health. In the case of Methylene Blue, its vibrant blue hue signifies more than just a dye; it's a chromatic link to potential health benefits.

Think of it as more than just a color. Methylene Blue's deep blue isn't just visually striking; it represents its multifaceted nature. This compound, originally known for its role as a dye, has expanded its repertoire to become a potential powerhouse in healthcare.

The chromatic connection becomes intriguing when we consider Methylene Blue's therapeutic properties. Its ability to combat diseases, act as an antioxidant, and play a role in neurological well-being adds depth to its vibrant color. It's not merely a pigment; it's a symbol of the complex interactions happening at the molecular level.

In exploring the chromatic aspect, we open a door to understanding how something as seemingly simple as color can be a visual cue to the compound's diverse applications. The colors we encounter hold the key to unlocking a spectrum of health benefits.

Methylene Blue isn't a newcomer in the world of health and well-being. With a history dating back almost two centuries, it has firmly established itself as a long-standing ally in the medical and wellness community. Notably, the World Health Organization recognizes its significance, listing Methylene Blue among its Essential Medicines. This acknowledgment speaks volumes about its unmatched importance and therapeutic value in various medical scenarios.

Despite its esteemed status, many of us tend to overlook Methylene Blue, especially as we navigate the challenges of age-related cognitive decline. Aging and certain lifestyle factors can lead to a decline in energy production within our brain cells, primarily driven by the inefficiency of our cellular powerhouses, the mitochondria.

This decline often manifests as reduced attention, memory lapses, and diminished mental clarity, typically surfacing in our 30s or 40s, depending on individual lifestyles.

Methylene Blue stands out due to its unique properties. It plays a crucial role in increasing oxygen delivery to brain cells, enhancing the efficiency of mitochondria. Beyond being a compound, Methylene Blue is a biological powerhouse. Its key feature lies in its ability to positively influence our biology at the cellular level, particularly in optimizing energy production by boosting mitochondrial efficiency a vital factor in sustaining and improving cognitive functions.

What makes Methylene Blue even more remarkable is its dual nature. On one hand, it boasts a rich historical legacy, and on the other, it remains a relatively undiscovered gem in the modern wellness landscape. It holds the potential to be a valuable asset for those seeking to optimize their brain health in the contemporary world of wellness.

Methylene blue works at a cellular level, specifically within the mitochondria, which are like the power stations in our cells that produce energy. Here, it influences energy production and can act like an antioxidant, helping to shield cells from oxidative stress. Since oxidative stress is linked to speeding up the aging process in people, methylene blue's antioxidant effects might have some anti-aging properties.

Also, methylene blue is a photosensitizer, meaning it becomes more active when exposed to certain types of light.

This light-activated property is used to treat donated blood products, as it's effective in killing some viruses like HIV and herpes. Because of its antiviral capabilities, there's been exploration into whether methylene blue could be a potential treatment for COVID-19.

Due to its potential in fighting viruses and its supposed anti-aging effects, some healthcare clinics offer methylene blue in different forms like skin creams and intravenous infusions. These are marketed to people who want to enhance their longevity, slow down aging, and prevent viral infections.

Conquering Cellular Distress

Combating Diseases and Battles Against COVID-19 and Alzheimer's

This compound called methylene blue that was initially made as a dye. But now, it's gaining a lot of attention in the health and wellness world because of its incredible effects on our bodies.

Let's talk about your mitochondria, these are like the power stations in your cells, making energy. Inside your mitochondria, there's a team of proteins called the electron transport chain. This chain is a pathway where electrons move around, releasing energy in the form of ATP (adenosine triphosphate).

Now, methylene blue does something cool. It acts like a redox agent or an electron carrier in this electron transport chain. In simple terms, it helps move electrons around, which leads to more ATP production, basically, the main energy currency for your cells. When your mitochondria work better, it boosts the overall energy in your cells and makes everything run more smoothly. That's how methylene blue helps optimize your cellular function and gives you a little energy boost.

Also, there are what we call the "Free radicals" which are like troublemakers in your body they're reactive and unstable molecules that go around stealing electrons from your healthy cells. Usually, your cells produce some free radicals as part of their normal activities. However, if you have a lot of inflammation going on, it can create even more of these troublemakers.

When there's too many free radicals hanging around, they start taking more electrons than they should. This steals from your cells and can cause damage called oxidative stress. And this is where methylene blue comes in like a superhero. It acts as an antioxidant, which means it neutralizes these troublesome free radicals and puts a stop to inflammation.

By doing this, methylene blue helps shield your cells from getting damaged by oxidative stress. It's like giving your cells some extra protection and lowering the risk of chronic diseases that often come from too much inflammation. Methylene blue gives your cells a power boost by making sure they get the essential nutrients and oxygen they need to work well. Here's how: Methylene blue adjusts the activity of something called nitric oxide synthase, which controls the production of nitric oxide (NO). Having the right levels of nitric oxide is crucial because it helps widen your blood vessels, a process known as vasodilation. When your blood vessels widen, it means that blood, nutrients, and oxygen can travel through your body more efficiently.

But that's not all, methylene blue also helps your cells use oxygen better. It's like turning up the efficiency dial on how your cells make use of the oxygen available to them. This double effect not only optimizes how your cells function at the tiny, cellular level but also gives a boost to your physical endurance and overall performance. It's like giving your body an extra edge to perform at its best.

Methylene blue falls into the category of nootropics, which are substances known to enhance brain performance. It achieves this in a few clear ways:

I. **Neurotransmitter Regulation:** Think of neurotransmitters as messengers in your brain that help different parts of your brain and your body communicate. Methylene blue steps in to improve both the release and reuptake of various neurotransmitters, including serotonin, dopamine, and norepinephrine.

II. **Monoamine Oxidase Inhibition:** After neurotransmitters do their job, they get broken down by an enzyme called monoamine oxidase. Methylene blue steps in here too, inhibiting these enzymes. This means more neurotransmitters are available, helping your brain work more effectively.

III. **Increased cGMP:** There's a special messenger molecule called cyclic guanosine monophosphate (cGMP), and it plays a crucial role in various functions in your body, especially in your brain.

Methylene blue gets your cells to produce more cGMP, raising the levels of this brain-boosting compound in your noggin.

When you put all of these effects together, you get an improvement in mood, focus, learning, and overall cognitive function. So, methylene blue is like a brain-boosting superhero with multiple powers to enhance how your brain works.

Neurodegeneration is like a gradual and often irreversible damage to your brain and nerve cells. Sometimes, it comes with the buildup of fiber deposits called amyloid proteins, making things even tougher for your brain to function smoothly. Methylene blue takes charge, supports and for the brain. And has been discovered to have neuroprotective powers, acting like a shield for your neurons against damage from harmful substances.

It supports the survival of nerve cells and plays a role in preventing neurodegenerative conditions. And that's not all, it also sticks to amyloid proteins, making them more stable and slowing down their buildup and deposition in the brain.

Alzheimer's Disease Solution

Methylene blue and its compounds are crucial because they hold potential benefits in managing Alzheimer's disease (AD). AD is a common disorder where cognitive abilities gradually decline, leading to severe dementia. With the aging population, the prevalence of AD is expected to increase.

In AD, there are identifiable intracellular tangles (neurofibrillary tissues or NFTs) and amyloid plaques in the brain. Methylene blue, often referred to as MB, is widely used in various fields like bacteriology, redox analysis, and medical treatment as an antiseptic for different ailments.

A groundbreaking study from 2016 reveals that as the brain ages, mitochondrial metabolism decreases. This decline might be a significant factor in many neurodegenerative diseases, including Alzheimer's. In simple terms, if your brain cells are metabolizing well, it's less likely to lead to dementia and other neurological diseases.

The health of your brain, including memory, concentration, and focus, depends on having enough energy in the form of adenosine triphosphate (ATP). As the production of energy within brain cells declines with age (known as the metabolic rate), so does your ability to think, remember, and communicate clearly.

One major reason why energy production slows down as we age is linked to nitric oxide. In medical training, nitric oxide has often been hailed as a "miracle molecule" for anti-aging, brain health, athletic performance, and overall well-being. However, recent evidence challenges this view.

Nitric oxide isn't a miracle molecule; it's a toxic free radical present in air pollution, and its role in dementia-related conditions like Alzheimer's is becoming clearer. In Alzheimer's patients, nitric oxide tends to gather around amyloid plaques in the brain, suggesting it could contribute to the brain cell death seen in dementia. This negative aspect of nitric oxide suggests that inhibitors like methylene blue might be highly effective in treating dementia. What ties nitric oxide to methylene blue?

Methylene blue happens to be one of the most powerful nitric oxide inhibitors known. It's like a tool that can significantly decrease the production of nitric oxide and clear existing nitric oxide from the blood and body. What makes methylene blue particularly intriguing is its ability to quickly accumulate in the brain, making it especially promising for various brain-related disorders, including dementia.

Scientists studying the brains of Alzheimer's patients over the years has noticed a common feature abnormally shaped TAU proteins or "neurofibrillary tangles" within brain cells called neurons. Methylene blue, a molecule originally developed as a fabric dye, could have a significant impact on resolving these issues.

In Alzheimer's disease, a key characteristic is the appearance of beta-amyloid plaques surrounding brain cells. Interestingly, methylene blue has been shown to prevent the formation of these plaques on the outside of neurons. Evidence suggests that methylene blue might address both primary hallmarks of Alzheimer's disease, neurofibrillary tangles and beta-amyloid plaques. Quite impressive for a compound initially designed for coloring fabric, how about, Alzheimer's patients outside the lab what is the impact of MB?

Methylene blue successfully halted Alzheimer's disease, or at the very least, it significantly improved its cognitive symptoms, which are the main focus in dealing with this type of dementia. Importantly, it was observed that drugs currently approved to manage Alzheimer's symptoms could hinder the positive effects of methylene blue when used together.

Now, when a therapy manages to stop cognitive decline by 83%, it raises the question of whether we can call it a cure. We need to be cautious and avoid making bold claims, but considering its effectiveness, methylene blue seems to be as close to a cure as we've seen for Alzheimer's disease. This groundbreaking drug, methylene blue, is a potent cognitive enhancer that has been scientifically proven to revive brain function in individuals with Alzheimer's.

The Anti-Aging Potentials of Methylene Blue and Skin Longevity

Analysis of gene expression revealed that treatment with Methylene Blue (MB) led to changes in the expression of certain extracellular matrix proteins in the skin. Notably, there was an increase in the levels of elastin and collagen 2A1, crucial components for maintaining healthy skin. This suggests that MB holds significant potential for skincare.

In the context of skin aging, oxidative stress plays a pivotal role, contributing to issues like wrinkles, pigmentation, and impaired wound healing. The use of antioxidants in skincare is widely acknowledged as an effective strategy to slow down the aging process. Methylene Blue, known for its traditional role as a mitochondrial-targeting antioxidant, demonstrated strong effectiveness in scavenging reactive oxygen species (ROS) in cultured human skin fibroblasts.

These fibroblasts were obtained from both healthy individuals and those with progeria, a genetic condition causing premature aging.

Comparing MB with other commonly used antioxidants, both general and mitochondrial-targeting, the results showed that MB outperformed in promoting the proliferation of skin fibroblasts and in delaying cellular senescence. This suggests that Methylene Blue could be a particularly effective option in skincare, not only for its antioxidant properties but also for its ability to enhance skin cell growth and resilience, offering a promising approach to combat the signs of aging.

The skin, being the largest and most visible organ in our body, undergoes changes as we age. Aged skin is characterized by the flattening of the dermal-epidermal junction and a general thinning of the extracellular matrix (ECM), which includes disorganized and reduced collagen and elastin.

There are two main types of skin aging, intrinsic and extrinsic. Intrinsic aging occurs naturally over time and is seen as fine wrinkles on dry skin.

Extrinsic aging is accelerated and results from exposure to sunlight and/or air pollution, leading to dry, rough, pigmented, and abraded skin, especially on the face and hands. Although these types of skin aging show different clinical features, both are influenced by oxidative damage caused by free radicals. Free radicals are molecules that can harm cells, and the skin experiences this damage partly due to them.

Maintaining a balance between the production of free radicals and the neutralization by antioxidants is how cells typically keep reactive oxygen species (ROS) at low levels. This balance is crucial for healthy skin, and disruptions in it contribute to the aging process, leading to the various changes observed in aged skin.

As we get older, a combination of increased accumulation of reactive oxygen species (ROS) and a decreased ability to clear these ROS leads to heightened oxidative stress. This oxidative stress causes damage to the large molecules in our organs. When the skin is regularly exposed to environmental stressors like UV radiation, smoke, and pollutants, it produces more free radicals, speeding up the aging process. The surplus of ROS reduces the production of collagen and increases its breakdown by triggering the expression of matrix metalloproteinase (MMP), ultimately altering the dermal matrix.

According to this ROS theory, an effective way to slow down skin aging is to provide antioxidants externally, such as through skincare products. These antioxidants can either suppress the production of free radicals or neutralize the excess ones, helping to maintain a healthier balance and preserve the skin's integrity over time.

Methylene blue, as an antioxidant, plays a vital role in counteracting free radicals, which helps diminish the appearance of fine lines and wrinkles while shielding cells from the damage caused by oxidative stress. Also, its anti-inflammatory properties work to reduce inflammation and minimize redness on the skin. What's more, methylene blue has a positive impact on collagen.

Collagen, a crucial structural protein, begins to decrease as early as our thirties. This protein acts like scaffolding in the skin, providing support to the outer layer. By the time we reach our mid-fifties, we've typically lost about 40% of our usual collagen levels, leading to sagging and wrinkles. Methylene blue comes into play by positively influencing fibroblasts, the cells responsible for collagen production. It achieves this by reducing reactive oxidative stress, a factor contributing to aging signs like wrinkles, slow wound healing, and pigmentation. In essence, methylene blue helps maintain skin firmness, decrease wrinkles, and promote overall skin health.

As cells age, they struggle to fend off free radicals due to a decline in the skin's usual supply of antioxidants. This decrease in antioxidants may vary from person to person, making the term "aging" quite broad. Interestingly, the need for antioxidants may not solely depend on chronological aging, especially since we now have a good understanding of pollutants and their impact on the skin.

Methylene blue stands out as a unique antioxidant with a specific focus on reactive oxygen species (ROS). It brings about lasting changes in cellular aging. What makes methylene blue distinctive is its ability to create permanent alterations within the cell by consistently keeping ROS levels low in all three major skin layers. This sets it apart as an effective agent in combating the aging process and maintaining skin health

How Methylene Blue Penetrates the Mitochondria and Modulate ROS in the Electron Transport Chain

Methylene blue possesses amphipathic properties, meaning it can dissolve in both oil and water, facilitating its penetration into intercellular compartments like mitochondria and lipid membranes. Unlike many antioxidants, such as vitamins, that are mostly either oil or water-soluble, methylene blue's amphipathic nature allows it to move in and out of mitochondria. This property is crucial as it enables methylene blue to regulate and mitigate the accumulation of reactive oxygen species (ROS)

in mitochondrial membranes. Unchecked ROS accumulation leads to both senescence and premature aging of the skin. The amphipathic characteristics of methylene blue, coupled with its low redox potential mentioned earlier, make it a self-generating antioxidant that can exist in both its oxidized and reduced forms simultaneously.

Its ability to accept electrons in the oxidized state or reject electrons in the reduced state allows it to enter the electron transport chain, helping to mitigate the buildup of free radicals. This, in turn, directly influences cellular functions and has the potential to alter or reverse the aging process.

Improving the hydration of aging skin brings noticeable benefits for us, such as smoother texture, a healthy glow, and often a reduction in fine wrinkles. As skin ages, it also becomes thinner over time due to a depletion of collagen and elastin. This thinning is likely a result of decreased enzymatic production in the extracellular matrix, coupled with an increase in reactive oxygen species (ROS) in the dermis.

This sets off a degenerative cycle that contributes to the aging process. After the age of forty, the production of both elastin and collagen drops rapidly, while ROS levels accumulate, intensifying the degenerative cycle. The elevated levels of ROS are likely a major contributor to both skin aging and related disorders.

Conditions like acne vulgaris contribute to the breakdown and production of collagen and elastin in the skin. Elastin is a crucial protein responsible for the pliability, resilience, and elasticity of the skin, promoting firmness and definition. Low levels of elastin and collagen result in sagging, wrinkle-prone skin. To counteract these effects, intrinsic antioxidant properties, such as those found in methylene blue, can be beneficial.

To further prove the great and important element in this dye, Researchers conducting skin tissue studies observed an increase in elastin fibers within the dermis after two weeks of treatment with methylene blue. This increase was associated with perceived anti-aging effects. The described properties of methylene blue, as outlined here, make it a versatile and potentially unique addition to the existing arsenal of antioxidants used in personal care products, complementing water-soluble vitamins, oil-soluble vitamins, and polyphenols.

Methylene Blue's Potential in Cancer Therapy

The role of Methylene Blue as an electron carrier and potential impact on cancer cells

Methylene Blue as a molecular courier within our cells, shuttling electrons in a dance crucial for generating cellular energy. This molecule doesn't merely carry electrons; it's a versatile player, gracefully transitioning between different states, orchestrating a delicate equilibrium.

Now, when it comes to cancer cells, Methylene Blue acts like a skilled infiltrator. It enters their mitochondria, the energy centers, and disrupts the normal flow of electron transfers. This disruption is strategic, nudging cancer cells towards programmed cell death while sparing healthy ones.

But Methylene Blue's does far more beyond that, Picture it as a key player in Photodynamic Therapy. When exposed to light, it transforms and releases reactive oxygen species, acting like precision-guided missiles against cancer cells.

Methylene Blue brings a significant advantage to cancer treatment through its unique ability to pinpoint and focus on cancer cells specifically. Unlike standard chemotherapy drugs that may harm both healthy and cancerous cells, Methylene Blue exclusively targets the cancer cells. This precision ensures that healthy cells remain untouched, potentially minimizing the common side effects associated with chemotherapy, like hair loss and nausea.

Moreover, Methylene Blue doesn't just stop at targeting cancer cells; it plays a collaborative role in other cancer treatments. For instance, it enhances the effectiveness of therapies like radiation treatment. By making cancer cells more sensitive to radiation, Methylene Blue has the potential to improve treatment outcomes and reduce the chances of cancer returning.

It's like having a strategic ally that not only takes on cancer directly but also amplifies the impact of other treatment approaches. The reason lies in its remarkable knack for zeroing in on cancer cells specifically. Imagine it as a precision tool that seeks out and hones in on these rogue cells.

Once Methylene Blue reaches these cancer cells, it doesn't just observe; it takes action. It puts the brakes on their growth, acting as a formidable opponent to tumor development. It's like a guardian preventing the expansion of these harmful clusters of cells.

Scientists have observed this effectiveness not just in one type of cancer but in several. Breast cancer, prostate cancer, and bladder cancer are among the varieties where Methylene Blue has showcased its potential. In essence, it's showing promise as a therapeutic ally in the battle against different forms of cancer. It's a bit like having a versatile warrior that can adapt its tactics to combat various foes on the cancer battlefield.

Methylene Blue's anticancer prowess involves a strategic approach, which zeroes in on the mitochondria within cancer cells. What happens is that Methylene Blue disrupts the electron transport chain within these cancer cell mitochondria. This disruption has a cascading effect, causing a decrease in ATP production, the energy currency of cells, and eventually triggering a process known as apoptosis in the cancer cells. In simpler terms, Methylene Blue interferes with the vital energy processes in cancer cells, prompting them to undergo a programmed cell death, a key factor in its anticancer effects.

"Apoptosis", is often referred to as programmed cell death, a natural and controlled process that occurs in multicellular organisms. In the context of cancer cells, apoptosis is a mechanism through which damaged or abnormal cells are directed to self-destruct.

In normal, healthy cells, apoptosis plays a crucial role in maintaining tissue homeostasis by eliminating cells that are no longer needed, damaged, or have undergone genetic mutations. It is a tightly regulated process that involves a series of molecular events leading to the orderly dismantling and removal of the cell.

In the case of cancer cells, one of the challenges is that they often evade apoptosis, allowing them to survive and proliferate uncontrollably. Methylene Blue, with its anticancer properties, is believed to induce apoptosis in cancer cells. Essentially, it triggers a process that instructs the cancer cells to undergo self-destruction, helping to control and eliminate these abnormal cells. This is a valuable aspect of anticancer treatments as it targets the cancer cells specifically, aiming to reduce the impact on healthy cells.

Enhanced Photodynamic Therapy efficacy of Methylene blue

Photodynamic therapy (PDT) is a method used to treat early proximal bronchial cancer during a flexible bronchoscopy. In this technique, a photosensitizer is excited by a specific wavelength and delivered into the bronchus near the tumor. PDT has become an important treatment approach for various cancers, as well as cardiovascular and ophthalmic diseases.

The process involves introducing light-sensitive molecules, known as photosensitizers, to target sites and then exposing them to a specific wavelength of light. When activated by light, these photosensitizers transfer their excess energy to surrounding oxygen, generating reactive oxygen species (ROS) like singlet oxygen ($1O2$) or free radicals. These ROS cause irreversible damage to diseased cells and tissues. PDT holds a significant value as a method to overcome multidrug resistance (MDR) since the cytotoxicity mechanism of photosensitizers differs from that of other chemotherapy agents. However, the widespread use of many photosensitizers has been hindered by significant side effects.

These include non-specific damage to normal tissues due to low selectivity for specific cells or tissues, environmental degradation, and hydrophobicity. To address these challenges, scientists have explored various biocompatible nanocarrier systems for delivering photosensitizers, including liposomes, polymeric micelles, and nanoparticles.

These nanocarriers play a crucial role in enhancing the uptake of photosensitizers into target sites, thereby reducing nonspecific damage to normal tissues caused by free photosensitizers furthermore, nanocarrier systems contribute to maintaining a stable aqueous dispersion of photosensitizers through surface modification and provide protection against environmental degradation.

Despite the numerous advantages offered by nanocarrier systems, their use has been somewhat limited, especially in the case of liposomes and micellar systems. This limitation stems from their lower drug loading capacity and the occurrence of severe side effects, such as anaphylactic shocks.

Methylene blue (MB) is a type of phenothiazinium photosensitizer which is used in various applications, including photodynamic therapy (PDT). Its ability to generate singlet oxygen ($1O_2$) efficiently in the therapeutic window (600–900 nm) makes it a promising choice for PDT. However, its clinical application has faced challenges due to its tendency to undergo rapid chemical changes when administered systemically.

In the biological environment, MB tends to undergo a chemical transformation by accepting electrons from nicotinamide adenine dinucleotide (NADH)/nicotinamide adenine dinucleotide phosphate (NADPH). This results in the formation of colorless leucomethylene blue, which lacks significant photodynamic activity.

One key factor in the reduction of MB is the presence of a transmembrane thiazine dye reductase at the cell surface. Cellular uptake of MB can further catalyze reduction with the help of NADH/NADPH dehydrogenases. The main challenge in using MB for PDT lies in formulating it into pharmaceutical preparations suitable for easy administration.

Consequently, there has been a focus on exploring biocompatible nanoparticles as effective carriers for encapsulating and delivering MB in PDT applications.

Calcium phosphate (CaP) materials have found widespread use in biomedical applications as effective carriers for drugs, mainly due to their excellent biocompatibility and bioactivity. Specifically, CaP nanoparticles incorporating photosensitizers have been synthesized with the aid of ionic polymers like poly(ethylene imine) and poly(styrene sulfonic acid).

These nanoparticles have shown notable phototoxicity against murine macrophages and bacteria. What sets CaP apart is its absorbability in specific cellular environments, such as endosomes/lysosomes, where it transforms into non-toxic ionic species. Utilizing controlled mineralization technology with self-assembled polymer templates has emerged as a successful approach to creating biocompatible and biodegradable nanocarriers for photosensitizers.

The primary aim of this study was to enhance the effectiveness of photodynamic therapy (PDT) by improving the biostability of methylene blue (MB).

This involves preventing environmental degradation and enzymatic reduction under biological conditions, thereby maximizing the potential of PDT. For a better understanding of all I have said in regards to the step-by-step explanation of enhanced photodynamic therapy (PDT) efficacy of methylene blue (MB) I have drafted a simple illustration:

Synthesis of CaP Nanoparticles: The process begins with the synthesis of calcium phosphate (CaP) nanoparticles, nanoparticles serve as carriers for the photosensitizer, in this case, (methylene blue) The synthesis is typically performed in the presence of ionic polymers like poly(ethylene imine) and poly(styrene sulfonic acid).

Incorporation of Photosensitizer: Methylene blue is incorporated into the CaP nanoparticles during their formation. This step ensures that the photosensitizer is efficiently encapsulated within the nanoparticles, promoting its stability and preventing premature activation.

Phototoxicity Testing: The resulting photosensitizer-loaded CaP nanoparticles are then subjected to testing for phototoxicity. This involves assessing their ability to induce cell death or damage to targeted cells, such as murine macrophages and bacteria. which helps to verify the effectiveness of the encapsulated methylene blue in causing cellular damage upon light exposure.

Specific Cellular Absorption: Calcium phosphate is known to be absorbable in specific cellular environments, particularly within endosomes/lysosomes. whose property is crucial for the targeted delivery of the encapsulated methylene blue to specific cellular compartments.

Utilization of Self-Assembled Polymer Templates: Controlled mineralization technology using self-assembled polymer templates is employed in the process.

This technique ensures the proper formation and stability of the CaP nanoparticles, enhancing their biocompatibility and biodegradability.

Prevention of Environmental Degradation: The study focuses on preventing environmental degradation of methylene blue and it involves protecting the photosensitizer from undergoing chemical alterations or degradation when exposed to external factors.

Enzymatic Reduction Prevention: Another critical aspect is preventing enzymatic reduction of methylene blue under biological conditions. This step is designed to maintain the stability of the encapsulated photosensitizer within the CaP nanoparticles, ensuring its efficacy during PDT.

Enhanced Photodynamic Therapy Efficacy: By optimizing the biostability of methylene blue through the use of CaP nanoparticles, the study aims to enhance the overall efficacy of photodynamic therapy. This involves maximizing the potential of methylene blue to generate reactive oxygen species upon light exposure, leading to improved outcomes in the treatment of various conditions, including cancers.

Combating Depression with Methylene Blue

Assessing the Effectiveness of Methylene Blue in Depression Treatment

Depression continues to be a widespread challenge, affecting millions worldwide and pushing the boundaries of available medical solutions. While traditional antidepressants have proven effective, there's room for improvement due to side effects and varying efficacy. In the field of psychiatry, methylene blue stands out with documented antidepressant, anxiolytic, and neuroprotective properties, observed in studies involving both animals and humans.

This substance has a stabilizing impact on mitochondrial function and notably controls the generation of reactive oxygen species, with its effects depending on dosage. These discoveries provide valuable insights, significantly advancing our understanding of the substance's potential in mental health applications.

Beyond psychiatry, methylene blue's influence extends from microbiology to pioneering the field of psychopharmacology. Its derivatives have inspired the creation of novel pharmacotherapeutic agents such as antimalarial medications, antihistamines, and the first generation of antipsychotic drugs. Contemporary research emphasizes methylene blue's potent metabolic-enhancing and antioxidant properties, which not only boost memory but also offer neuroprotection.

In the intricate web of mood disorders, it's challenging to pinpoint a single neurotransmitter system or signaling process as the definitive cause. Recognizing this complexity has sparked interest in multi-target drugs for treating such conditions. Methylene blue, with its diverse range of biological mechanisms, enters this arena. It modulates redox processes and mitochondrial functions, inhibits monoamine oxidase A (MAO-A), and influences signal transduction, all relevant aspects for neuropsychiatry.

Early reports by Narsapur and Naylor suggested the potential effectiveness of methylene blue in treating both phases of manic-depressive psychosis, especially when traditional therapies fell short. Studies indicated improvement in patients receiving both intravenous and oral methylene blue. A two-year double-blind crossover trial demonstrated reduced depression levels with an increased daily dose of the compound. Further research confirmed substantial positive effects of methylene blue on symptoms of depression and anxiety in patients with bipolar disorder. Importantly, there were no signs of serotonergic toxicity, even at a dosage of 195 mg.

Methylene blue, known for its strong neuroprotective and anti-inflammatory properties, could be a crucial player in treating various neurodegenerative disorders. To make the most of its pharmacological power, compounded capsules are an ideal form. They provide stability, allow precise dosages customized to individual requirements, mask the compound's unpleasant taste, and offer convenient portability.

Patients with bipolar disorder often find relief from mood-stabilizing treatments, but full remission of affective symptoms remains a challenge. Persistent low-grade depression, mood cycling, and anxiety are frequent, lasting a significant portion of the time and increasing the risk of relapse and ongoing disability. Additionally, cognitive changes, resistant to standard long-term treatments, contribute to disability. Many see bipolar disorder as a progressive condition, leading to cognitive impairment and grey matter loss in specific brain regions.

Now let's talk about the scientific evidence supporting Methylene Blue's antidepressant properties. It's crucial to understand the mechanisms through which this compound may alleviate depressive symptoms.

Methylene Blue has been a subject of both animal and human studies, revealing its antidepressant, anxiolytic, and neuroprotective properties. These effects are not merely anecdotal; they've been documented in rigorous scientific investigations. Imagine it as a versatile tool, not just targeting one aspect but wielding a holistic influence on our mental well-being

The chemistry behind its antidepressant prowess, Methylene Blue plays a pivotal role in modulating redox processes. What does that mean, you ask? Well, it helps balance the oxidation-reduction reactions in our cells, contributing to the stability of our cellular environment. Picture it as an orchestra conductor, orchestrating harmony in the symphony of our cellular processes.

Methylene Blue influences mitochondrial functions. Mitochondria are the powerhouses of our cells, and their optimal function is crucial for maintaining a healthy mental state. By interacting with these cellular energy hubs, Methylene Blue contributes to the overall stability of our mental processes.

Now, here comes an intriguing aspect, Methylene Blue inhibits monoamine oxidase A (MAO-A). Think of MAO-A as a regulator in the neurotransmitter world. By inhibiting it, Methylene Blue helps maintain the delicate balance of neurotransmitters like serotonin, dopamine, and norepinephrine. It's like ensuring the smooth flow of communication in the intricate network of our brain.

By inhibiting MAO-A, Methylene Blue extends the duration of these neurotransmitters' presence, fostering a more sustained and balanced neuronal communication. It's like extending the life of messengers in a vital communication network, promoting stability in our mental landscape.

Moreover, Methylene Blue influences signal transduction. This refers to the transmission of signals within our cells. By modulating these signaling pathways, Methylene Blue can impact various cellular responses, including those related to mood and mental well-being.

In the early days of psychopharmacology, Methylene Blue derivatives paved the way for novel pharmacotherapeutic agents. These derivatives inspired the synthesis of medications, ranging from antimalarials to antipsychotic drugs. So, you can see, Methylene Blue's impact spans from the microscopic world of cells to the broader field of psychiatry.

the Methylene Blue's impact on redox processes is akin to maintaining a delicate equilibrium in a dynamic system. It acts as a scavenger, intercepting and neutralizing harmful reactive oxygen species (ROS) that can disrupt cellular balance. By doing so, it safeguards against oxidative stress, a known contributor to depressive symptoms.

Methylene Blue exhibits a profound influence. It interacts with the electron transport chain, a crucial part of mitochondrial function. This interaction not only enhances energy production but also contributes to the stability of cellular processes reliant on this energy. Imagine it as a catalyst, boosting the power output of our cellular engines and ensuring a steady supply of energy for optimal mental function.

The landscape of Methylene Blue's antidepressant mechanisms, is a versatile agent operating at the crossroads of cellular chemistry. Its actions span from maintaining cellular balance to fine-tuning neurotransmitter dynamics and orchestrating intricate signaling pathways. This multifaceted approach aligns with the complexity of depressive disorders, offering a promising avenue for those seeking relief from the burdens of mood disorders.

In essence, Methylene Blue doesn't just touch the surface; it intricately intertwines with the molecular intricacies of our cells, offering a potential key to unlocking the mysteries of depression and paving the way for innovative approaches in mental health therapeutics

Heart Disease and Methylene Blue

Methylene Blue positive impact on cardiovascular health and potential benefits

As we know, postoperative hypotension is a common conundrum in the aftermath of cardiac surgery. The triumvirate of hemodynamic disorders, hypovolemia, vasoplegia, and heart failure takes center stage, often leading to episodes of hypotension associated with unfavorable outcomes.

Vasoplegic syndrome (VS), a notable complication post-cardiopulmonary bypass, adds another layer of complexity, characterized by severe hypotension, altered cardiac outputs, and diminished systemic vascular resistance.

Among them, vasoplegia poses a significant challenge as it shows minimal responsiveness to common vasopressors like norepinephrine. This condition, known as cardiac vasoplegic syndrome (CVS), is linked to higher mortality rates.

Vasoplegic syndrome (VS) is a well-recognized complication of cardiopulmonary bypass (CPB), occurring in 5% to 25% of cases. It manifests with substantial hypotension, normal or high cardiac outputs, low systemic vascular resistance (SVR), and an increased need for fluids and vasopressors during or after CPB. Patients experiencing VS face elevated risks of death and other major complications post-cardiac surgery.

The standard approach to managing cardiac vasoplegic syndrome (CVS) involves the administration of fluids and catecholamines, like norepinephrine. The development of vasoplegia in this context is driven by the activation of various systems, including contact, coagulation, and complement systems, as well as the activation of leukocytes, platelets, and endothelial cells.

This cascade disrupts the regulation of vascular tone after cardiac surgery, leading to vasoplegia. Several risk factors have been identified to predict the occurrence of vasoplegia. While treatment primarily relies on vasopressors, some cases may not respond well to these medications, resulting in refractory hypotension.

Methylene Blue, a potential protagonist in this cardiovascular saga. Conventional treatment involves the administration of fluids and catecholamines, like norepinephrine. However, Methylene Blue emerges as an alternative, aiming to modulate the intricate interplay of contact, coagulation, and complement systems, along with leukocytes, platelets, and endothelial cells, that seeks to restore the delicate balance of vascular tone, a pivotal factor in postcardiac surgery vasoplegia.

Catecholamines, commonly used in treatment, come with notable side effects like increased myocardial oxygen consumption, arrhythmias, and decreased blood flow to organs. To mitigate these risks, an additional treatment to reduce the need for catecholamines becomes crucial. The overarching goal in cardiovascular care is to maintain proper systemic blood flow and perfusion pressure for organ homeostasis.

Striking the right balance between vasoconstriction and vasodilation is essential, especially when pathological conditions tip the scale toward a vasodilatory state, potentially compromising organ perfusion.

Why Methylene Blue, you may wonder? Unlike its catecholamine counterparts, Methylene Blue seeks to mitigate side effects such as increased oxygen consumption and arrhythmias. The cardiovascular system's primary goal is maintaining adequate blood flow and perfusion pressure, and Methylene Blue aids in achieving this delicate equilibrium between vasoconstriction and vasodilation

In conditions like distributive shock leading to vasoplegia, Methylene Blue is a stalwart. It tackles the multifaceted pathophysiology, offering a non-catecholaminergic approach. Its ability to increase mean arterial pressure without serious adverse events, as evidenced in studies, positions it as a potential panacea for patients grappling with cardiac vasoplegic syndrome.

During cardiac surgery, the production of reactive oxygen species (ROS) can contribute to complications. Methylene Blue's role as an antioxidant is crucial. It helps neutralize ROS, preventing oxidative stress-related damage. This antioxidant property contributes to the overall protection of the cardiovascular system, supporting a healthier recovery process, Catecholamines, often used in postoperative care, can have drawbacks.

Methylene Blue, by reducing catecholamine stress, employs a strategy known as decatecholaminisation which helps in preventing side effects associated with catecholamines but also contributes to improved survival rates in patients experiencing cardiac vasoplegic syndrome.

Beyond immediate recovery, Methylene Blue's neuroprotective properties have implications for long-term cognitive health. Postoperative complications, including those related to hypotension, can sometimes impact cognitive function. Methylene Blue, with its multifaceted benefits offer a protective shield against such cognitive consequences.

The pathophysiology of vasoplegia is intricate, involving the activation of intrinsic vasodilatory pathways and a pathological insensitivity to vasopressors. In this state, the body struggles to achieve sufficient end-organ perfusion pressure due to a lack of vascular tone, even with adequate or elevated cardiac output (CO). Importantly, patients in vasoplegic states show minimal responsiveness to pharmacological agents designed to increase systemic vascular resistance (SVR). Regardless of the specific cause, mortality rates in patients with vasoplegia can be alarmingly high, reaching up to 50%. Determining the optimal treatment strategy remains a point of controversy.

Concerns linger regarding the emphasis on restoring macrocirculatory parameters through vasoconstrictors, as the primary goal should be optimizing microcirculatory function. Methylene blue (MB), a non-catecholaminergic agent, has emerged as a therapeutic alternative or adjuvant to classic vasoplegic syndrome therapies.

57

It has demonstrated a statistically significant increase in mean arterial pressure (MAP) without causing serious adverse events, as highlighted in a meta-analysis of five randomized controlled trials. One notable benefit of MB is its ability to reduce catecholamine stress in critically ill patients, a phenomenon known as decatecholaminization.

This effect may contribute to improved survival in individuals with cardiac vasoplegic syndrome (CVS).

The Cardiovascular Epicenter

At the core of Methylene Blue's prowess lies its ability to navigate the intricate web of cardiovascular challenges. Imagine our cardiovascular system as a symphony, with each component playing a crucial role. Methylene Blue steps onto this stage as a conductor, orchestrating a harmonious balance.

let's take the cardiovascular system as a grand symphony, where the heart, blood vessels, and various components perform distinct roles. This symphony, when well-coordinated, ensures the smooth circulation of blood, maintaining life's rhythm. However, disruptions, like those encountered post-cardiac surgery, can introduce discord.

And this is where Methylene Blue takes center stage. Think of it as the conductor of this intricate symphony. With its unique properties, Methylene Blue doesn't merely address a single instrument's issue; it harmonizes the entire orchestra. It navigates through the complexity, guiding each component to play in unison, creating a balanced and melodious composition.

In cardiovascular challenges, balance is key. Blood vessels need to maintain tone, the heart must pump effectively, and systemic pressures should align. Methylene Blue, like a skilled conductor, ensures this delicate equilibrium. It modulates redox processes, influences mitochondrial functions, and inhibits pathways that may lead to complications, fostering a cardiovascular harmony.

The cardiovascular symphony isn't always straightforward. Post-cardiac surgery, disturbances in vascular tone and hemodynamics can disrupt the musical flow. Methylene Blue steps in as the knowledgeable conductor, guiding the ensemble through the intricacies. It addresses not only the immediate issues but also anticipates potential challenges, ensuring a seamless performance.

When the cardiovascular system encounters disruptions, Methylene Blue introduces a new melody, a melody of recovery. It doesn't overpower or drown out the existing instruments; instead, it enhances their capabilities, allowing the symphony to regain its original rhythm. This melody signifies not just treatment but a pathway to restoration and healing.

In essence, Methylene Blue's role in the cardiovascular symphony is that of a conductor who understands the intricacies, anticipates challenges, and ensures that each component plays its part harmoniously.

Practical Applications and Administration of Methylene Blue in Healthcare

Methylene Blue is not confined to a single medical niche. It spans a wide spectrum of applications, ranging from antimicrobial solutions to treatments for conditions like Alzheimer's, autism, heart disease, and cancer. One standout feature is its potent antimicrobial properties. Methylene Blue has demonstrated effectiveness against various pathogens, making it a valuable tool in combating infections.

Its role in addressing mitochondrial dysfunction is another highlight. Understanding how it interacts with cellular energy production sheds light on its potential in conditions related to energy imbalance. Methylene Blue's neuroprotective effects have garnered attention in the context of neurodegenerative disorders. This includes Alzheimer's and autism, where its impact on brain health is under exploration.

n the cardiovascular realm, Methylene Blue's ability to navigate complex hemodynamic challenges after cardiac surgery positions it as a valuable asset, showcasing its adaptability in critical medical scenarios. Its potential in cancer therapy introduces yet another dimension. Methylene Blue's impact on cancer cells and its ability to selectively target them open avenues for innovative approaches in cancer treatment.

The fact that Methylene Blue continues to be a subject of active research underscores its evolving role. Ongoing studies explore new dimensions of its applications, adding to the excitement surrounding its versatility. What makes Methylene Blue particularly intriguing is its ability to contribute to a more holistic healthcare approach. Its applications span across various medical domains, offering a multifaceted tool for healthcare professionals

Ultimately, understanding the versatility of Methylene Blue is of great importance for healthcare practitioners seeking effective, targeted, and patient-centric solutions. It opens avenues for personalized treatment strategies targeted towards individual health needs.

Recently an experiment was conducted in the to examine the value of this methylene blue on healthcare, and the results we got was astonishing, I will do my best to explain in the simplest way so we can all be on the same page.

Methylene Blue's Potential for Pain Relief Unveiled

Growing evidence suggests that Methylene Blue (MB) does more than we might think, it's not just a dye! In fact, it has the ability to tackle abnormal vasodilation and even help with pain relief. Some smart doctors started injecting MB into worn-out disks in the spine to ease the pain for folks dealing with chronic discogenic low back pain (CDLBP), and the results were pretty amazing.

For conditions like osteoarthritis and colitis, MB steps in as a pain-relief superhero by calming down inflammation. It does this by putting a brake on the production of nitric oxide, which is a troublemaker causing inflammation. But here's the interesting part even with these cool pain-relief powers, MB hasn't gotten much attention from the public. So, let's dig into how MB works its magic on pain. There are three main things it does: fights inflammation, reduces sodium currents (like turning down an electrical switch), and acts on the nerves. these actions come together to make MB a potential game-changer for pain relief.

But, and there's always a "but," right? We need to talk about some debates around using MB for CDLBP. Not everyone agrees on how effective it is, and there are also concerns about its safety in certain situations. This book aims to be the first to really break down how MB helps with pain, giving us a fresh perspective on it as a pain-relief solution.

Let's get into why inflammation matters when it comes to pain. Inflammation is like a sidekick to pain; it often triggers responses in our nerves that make us feel pain. MB does its thing by directly telling endothelial NOS (eNOS) to chill out, which is a big deal because eNOS is a troublemaker that leads to nitric oxide. And we know nitric oxide is not our friend in this story. MB also throws a wrench into the machinery that converts guanosine triphosphate (GTP) into cyclic guanosine monophosphate (cGMP) in our muscles, leading to a helpful tightening of the blood vessels.

In a nutshell, MB might be our new pain-relief buddy by calming down inflammation and tweaking how our nerves respond. It's like a behind-the-scenes hero working to make us feel better. Exciting stuff, right?

Methylene Blue (MB) fights pain on two fronts: it's a pro at calming inflammation, and it knows how to soothe our nerves. When things go haywire in our body, and tissues get injured, a troublemaker called iNOS steps in. It's like an inflammatory mediator causing chaos. MB steps in and says,

66

"Hold up, let's cool it down." MB puts a stop to iNOS and also interferes with a big player called NF-κB, which is like a boss orchestrating the inflammatory response.

By doing this, MB disrupts the whole inflammatory signaling process, preventing a cascade of events that lead to more inflammation and cell damage.

Nerve injuries activate something called NMDA receptors, which are like gatekeepers for pain signals. They let in a bunch of calcium, setting off a chain reaction that leads to persistent pain. MB blocks the activation of nNOS, another troublemaker, and also calms down the production of a signaling molecule called cGMP in doing this, MB puts the brakes on the whole process that leads to long-term pain and hypersensitivity. It's like telling the nerves to take a chill pill.

In the world of our body's pathways, there's a troublemaker called NO (Nitric Oxide). Which act as a mediator that stirs up inflammation, causing all sorts of problems. MB knows that NO is a key player in inflammation, so it targets a specific pathway called iNOS/NO. This pathway usually activates NF-κB, a big boss that promotes inflammation and can even cause cell death.

MB shows its skills. It's like a peacekeeper that inhibits the iNOS/NO pathway, preventing the activation of NF-κB. Think of NF-κB as the conductor of an inflammatory orchestra, making a lot of noise and MB the boss that steps in and turns down the volume. There's also a good guy named Sirt1, which normally keeps NF-κB and another troublemaker, p53, in check. But when iNOS/NO is in action, Sirt1 gets sidelined. MB changes the game by keeping iNOS in check, directly putting a lid on inflammation and also stopping NF-κB from creating chaos.

Methylene Blue's Cartilage Saver and Gut Guardian

In our body's cartilage (that stuff keeping our joints happy), Methylene Blue (MB) does some serious work for it. Imagine our cartilage as a precious structure that needs protection. When things go wrong and inflammation kicks in, it lead to the breakdown of this cartilage.

In human cartilage, MB acts like a shield, reducing the accumulation of a troublemaker NO (Nitric Oxide) and putting a cap on iNOS (another culprit causing inflammation and boosts the receptors for Transforming Growth Factor Beta (TGF-β), which is like a superhero for cartilage, helping in its repair and synthesis. The result? Cartilage breakdown is prevented, and the proteoglycan (cartilage's best friend) stays intact and healthy.

On the other hand, Opioids, like morphine, are great in the pain-relief world. They work by connecting with opioid receptors (ORs) and pulling off a clever move to reduce pain signals turning down the volume on those pesky pain messages.

But, here's the catch. Opioids, while excellent at their job, have some not-so-cool side effects. They can lead to addiction and cause problems. Morphine, for example, might throw a bit of a party in your body, inviting inflammatory troublemakers like IL-1β, IL-6, and TNF-α. This inflammation can cause some serious issues and even harm your nerves, whereas MB shows a superior confidence in toning down the action of something called nNOS, which is like a switch for inflammation. So, just like turning down the volume on pain, MB can do the same for inflammation.

In a real-life scenario, there are reports that says people dealing with stubborn mouth pain found relief with MB. Those using MB needed way less morphine to tackle their pain.

How does Methylene Blue effect a positive change in Pain Relief in relation to the ATP Receptor, well the stars of our tale is the Purinergic P2X receptor subtypes. These receptors are like little sensors that can cause inflammation and pain. They get activated when they bind with a molecule called adenosine $5'$ - triphosphate (ATP).

these receptors act as tiny channels that let different ions (like $K+$, $Na+$, and $Ca2+$) through. When they open, they can change the charge of neurons, setting off a chain reaction that activates various signaling pathways.

In our nerve world (specifically in the dorsal root ganglion or DRG), there are two key factor, P2X3 and P2X2/3, which steals the spotlight. They're like messengers stationed in small nerve fibers, and their job is crucial "transmitting pain signals".

It turns out that MB has a close connection with the events orchestrated by these P2X receptors. It's like MB is part of the pain-relief orchestra, influencing how these receptors work.

Forms and Dosages

When I say form and dosages, I'm referring to the different physical types or presentations in which a medication is available. For Methylene Blue, it can come in various forms, such as:

> **Oral Tablets or Pills:** Methylene Blue can be formulated into solid tablets or pills for oral consumption. This is a common form for medications that need to be ingested.

➤ **Solution or Liquid Form:** Methylene Blue can also be prepared as a liquid solution. This form is often used for injections, but there are oral liquid formulations as well.

➤ **Topical Applications:** In some cases, Methylene Blue are included in creams, gels, or other topical formulations. This is when the medication is applied directly to the skin.

Dosage is the amount or concentration of the medication that is administered to a patient. Dosages can vary based on factors like the patient's age, weight, the severity of the condition, and the form of the medication:

➤ **Oral Dosages:** If it's in tablet form for oral consumption, the dosage will be specified in terms of milligrams (mg) or micrograms (mcg) per tablet. The dosage will vary based on the condition being treated.

➤ **Injectable Dosages:** If Methylene Blue is administered through injections, the dosage will be determined by the healthcare provider based on the condition and diagnoses and patient's needs. This could be specified in milligrams or other units depending on the concentration of the solution.

➤ **Topical Dosages:** For topical applications, dosages are expressed in terms of the amount of Methylene Blue per unit of the topical product.

Administration Protocols and Considerations

I always advise against self-medication, and if you must, if need be (in the case of an emergency), there are critical administration protocols and considerations to bear in mind, especially with a medication like Methylene Blue.

First and foremost, the **route of administration** plays a pivotal role. If Methylene Blue is prescribed in a tablet or liquid form for oral intake, it is crucial to follow the prescribed dosage and take it as directed. This ensures that the medication is absorbed properly through the digestive system.

In emergency situations or specific medical procedures, healthcare providers might opt for the **intravenous (IV) route**, where Methylene Blue is directly infused into the bloodstream. This method allows for a rapid and controlled delivery of the medication.

For certain skin conditions or localized treatments, a topical application may be recommended. This involves applying Methylene Blue directly to the affected area, ensuring targeted therapeutic effects.

Additionally, in some cases, an **intramuscular (IM) injection** may be administered, particularly if oral intake is not feasible.

Dosage timing is another critical factor. Always adhere to the prescribed frequency and timing of Methylene Blue administration. Whether it's a daily oral dose, an IV infusion, or a one-time injection, **consistency** is key to achieving the desired therapeutic effects

Special instructions, if any, should not be overlooked. This could include taking Methylene Blue with or without food, avoiding specific substances that may interact adversely, or following any additional guidelines provided by the healthcare provider.

Consideration of patient characteristics is paramount. Factors such as age, weight, overall health, and the specific medical condition being treated influence the appropriate dosage and route of administration.

Always be vigilant about potential **interactions.** Methylene Blue may interact with other medications or substances, and understanding these interactions is crucial to avoid adverse effects.

Regular **monitoring** is essential. Healthcare providers will assess how the patient responds to the medication, monitoring for any side effects and adjusting the dosage if necessary.

Contraindications must be taken into account. In situations where Methylene Blue may pose risks, alternative treatments or precautions should be explored.

Proper **storage and stability** are also considerations. Following recommended storage conditions, such as temperature and protection from light, ensures the medication remains effective.

Patient education is a fundamental aspect. Providing clear information on how to take the medication, potential side effects, and what steps to take in case of missed doses or adverse reactions empowers the patient in their treatment.

while self-medication is discouraged, and I still think its best, understanding these administration protocols and considerations is vital for anyone prescribed Methylene Blue. It ensures the safe and effective use of this medication in various therapeutic contexts.

Side Effects of Methylene Blue

Intravenous route (Solution)

Too much of anything is bad, this holds true in many aspects of life, including the use of medications or substances. It emphasizes the importance of moderation and balance. Even with substances that may have potential benefits, excessive use or misuse can lead to adverse effects. In the case of Methylene Blue or any other medication, it's vital to follow prescribed doses, adhere to recommended guidelines, and consult with healthcare professionals to ensure safety and efficacy.

Health decisions should always be made with careful consideration of individual factors, and seeking professional advice is also a major key part of maintaining well-being. the risk of side effects increases with higher

Combining methylene blue with certain medications can lead to a severe condition known as serotonin syndrome, which can be serious or fatal. It's crucial to avoid using methylene blue together with drugs that affect serotonin levels, such as selective serotonin reuptake inhibitors (SSRIs), serotonin and norepinephrine reuptake inhibitors (SNRIs), and monoamine oxidase inhibitors. This caution is important to prevent the risk of harmful interactions and ensure safety in medication use.

The dosage for Methylene Blue is typically 0.045 to 0.09 mL per pound of body weight. It's important to inform your doctor about all the medications you are taking, as Methylene Blue may interact with acetazolamide, antacids, sodium bicarbonate, or diuretics (water pills).

If you are pregnant, there may be potential harm to the fetus, although, in some cases, the medication might still be used under your doctor's evaluation of safety. It's crucial to discuss your pregnancy with your doctor. It's unclear whether Methylene Blue passes into breast milk or poses a risk to a nursing baby. If you are breastfeeding, consult your doctor before continuing. Always follow your healthcare provider's advice for a safe and effective use of the medication. With that being said, there are list of may or may-not be side effect I have put together, these side effects are rare, and their occurrence is not well-documented:

i. Agitation
ii. Bluish-colored lips, fingernails, or palms
iii. Chest tightness
iv. Confusion
v. Cough
vi. Dark urine
vii. Diarrhea
viii. Difficulty breathing
ix. Difficulty swallowing
x. Dizziness or lightheadedness
xi. Fast heartbeat
xii. Fever
xiii. Headache
xiv. Hives or welts, itching, or skin rash

xv. Large, hive-like swelling on the face, eyelids, lips, tongue, throat, hands, legs, feet, or sex organs

xvi. Overactive reflexes

xvii. Pale skin

xviii. Poor coordination

xix. Rapid heart rate

xx. Redness of the skin

xxi. Restlessness

xxii. Shivering

xxiii. Sore throat

xxiv. Sweating

xxv. Talking or acting with excitement you cannot control

xxvi. Trembling or shaking

xxvii. Twitching

xxviii. Unusual bleeding or bruising

xxix. Unusual tiredness or weakness.